I0421609

Legal & Disclaimer

The information contained in this book is not designed to replace or take the place of any form of medication or professional medical advice. The information in this book has been provided for educational and entertainment purposes only.

The information contained in this book has been compiled from sources deemed reliable, and it is accurate to the best of the Author's knowledge. However, the Author cannot guarantee its accuracy and validity so cannot be held liable for any errors or omissions. Changes are periodically made to this book. You must consult your doctor or get professional medical advice before using any of the suggested remedies, techniques, or information in this book.

Upon using the information contained in this book, you agree to hold harmless the Author from and against any damages, costs and expenses, including any legal fees, potentially resulting from the application of any of the information provided by this guide. This disclaimer applies to any damages or injury caused by the use and application, whether directly or indirectly, of any advice or information presented, whether for breach of contract, tort, negligence, personal injury, criminal intent, or under any other cause of action.

You agree to accept all the risks of using the information presented inside this book. You need to consult a professional medical practitioner in order to ensure you are both able & healthy enough to participate in this program.

Contents

Introduction

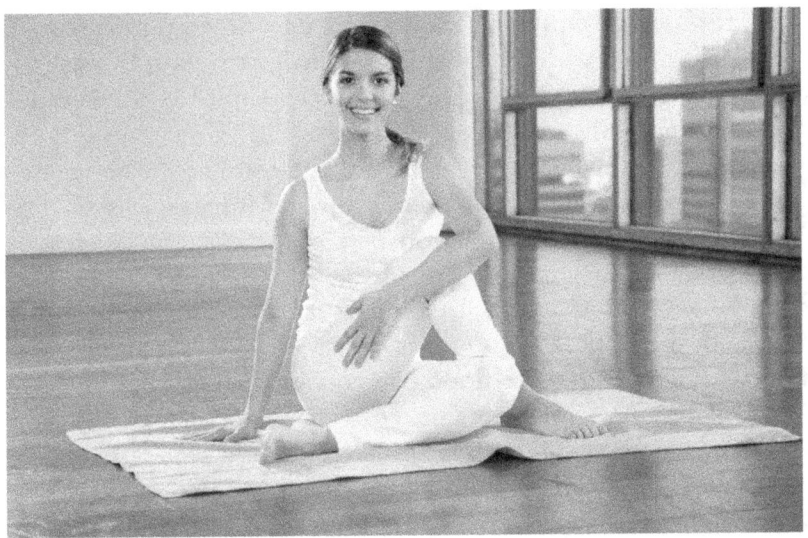

Thank you for downloading this yoga book.

Of all the wellness guides available, one of the most widely desired are those on weight loss. Keeping and maintaining a good body shape seems essential for projecting a healthy and professional body image nowadays; obesity has been one of the most widespread health concerns in developed countries and is also one of the major causes leading to other health issues like diabetes, high blood pressure and heart ailments.

A Simpler, Easier and Faster Way to Weight Loss, Stress Relief, Heal Your Body and Find Inner Peace and Balance.

In the past few decades, the practice of yoga has gained popularity. However, most of the widely available knowledge may not be easy to follow. The often impossible-looking postures seem forbidding and one often wonders if its benefits are effective. The good news is that there is a yoga fit for everyone! One of the interesting facts about the practice of yoga is that almost anyone can master it regardless of gender, age, race or physical limitations!

This book is unique in the sense that the explanations are kept simple with minimum theoretical jargon. It is out of the ordinary, unlike the run-of-the-mill guides that are flooding cyberspace. Through this book you will enter the amazing world of yoga. You will gain insight on how to get started and the things to keep in mind while practicing yoga. These are important as they will help bring overall improvements in your life not only to help in losing weight but also for finding inner peace. Tips on how to maximize the benefits of simple postures are given in this book. All you need is 30 minutes a day for maximized results!

Congratulate yourself on your first step towards total happiness.

A Simpler, Easier and Faster Way to Weight Loss, Stress Relief, Heal Your Body and Find Inner Peace and Balance.

Essential Benefits of Yoga for Everyone

Before we open the doors to the world of yoga for weight loss, let us take a brief glimpse into the past. This is essential because by learning about the history of yoga, one can appreciate why this ancient practice has withstood the test of time.

History in Brief

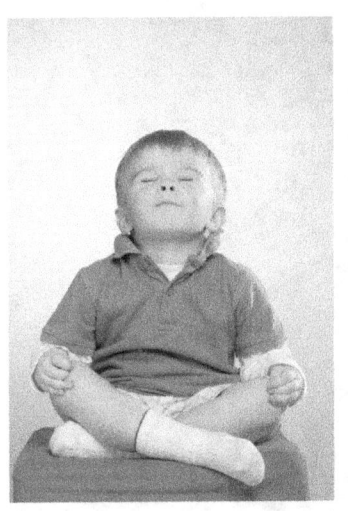

The word "yoga" is a Sanskrit word meaning "union." The practice of yoga involves a harmonious union of mind, body and spirit. There is great emphasis on a proper breathing technique as breath is the tool to connect these three aspects.

Over the years, it developed into a more ritualistic way of life followed by a more spiritual internalization of the principles of yoga. Patanjali, in the second century B.C., is the first to be credited with putting them down as scriptures, some of which have influenced yoga as we know it today.

Gradually, the forms of practice were modified by various yoga masters and came to involve the body-centered practices as is popular in modern times. Despite the various methods, the purpose remains fairly the same: to explore the physical and spiritual connection for our betterment.

5

Contrary to some opinions, yoga is not based on any religion. Rather, it is a way of living which has been perfected over thousands of years. The regular and correct practice of yoga has many benefits which is why it has gained popularity in the West. Hence, a brief overview is in order.

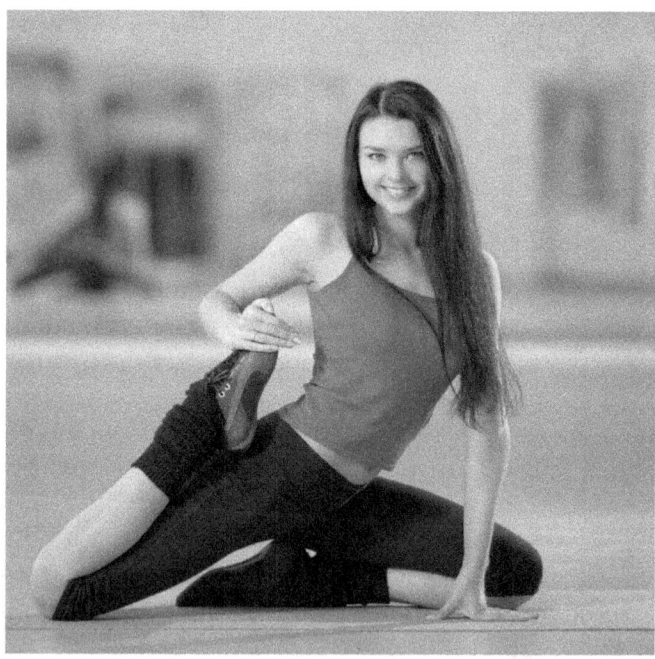

Physical Benefits of Yoga

Let's see how the practice of yoga will help. The immediate benefits one experiences are physical.

1)   Flexibility

The very first impression a layman gets at the thought of yoga is about having to touch one's toes. This is not far from the truth; however, this is not the entire truth. During the early days of your practice, you may experience slight soreness. This is especially true if you have not been exercising on a regular basis. Not to worry, the stiffness will disappear within a few days; you will feel more flexibility and the soreness will soon vanish giving rise to rejuvenated muscles and joints. This is also true with the body postures. You will realize that you can now hold on to the posture slightly longer and notice the discomfort gradually reducing. This incredible feeling will motivate you to look forward to more benefits of yoga.

2)   Better health

The practice of yoga involves control and exercise of the muscles.

This, along with proper control over breathing and posture, helps keep the internal organs in good condition. It promotes healing from within. The use of breathing to reach life-giving oxygen to the cells of the body helps to keep them healthy and consequently delay the onset of aging.

During metabolism, a high amount of toxins is produced within the body. The accumulation of toxins causes deterioration in the quality and functioning of the organs of the human body. Yoga helps flush out toxins and keeps you energized.

•   Improves arthritis: Guided treatment with yoga benefits arthritis and reduces back pain. Certain postures strengthen the muscles of the back and increase lubrication of joints. It is best to learn these exercises under supervision as the incorrect technique may result in aggravation of the condition.

•   Improves asthma and other respiratory ailments: patients with respiratory problems have shown positive changes in their condition with practices in control of breath and concentration. It can also aid improvement lung efficiency.

•   Biochemical changes are brought about due to the activation of certain glands. This also helps in controlling those glands, the imbalance of which can lead to diabetes and high cholesterol levels.

Mental Benefits of Yoga

The essence of yoga is the unity of mind and body. The aim is to achieve a balanced state. The mental state of a person greatly influences his or her physiology and vice versa.

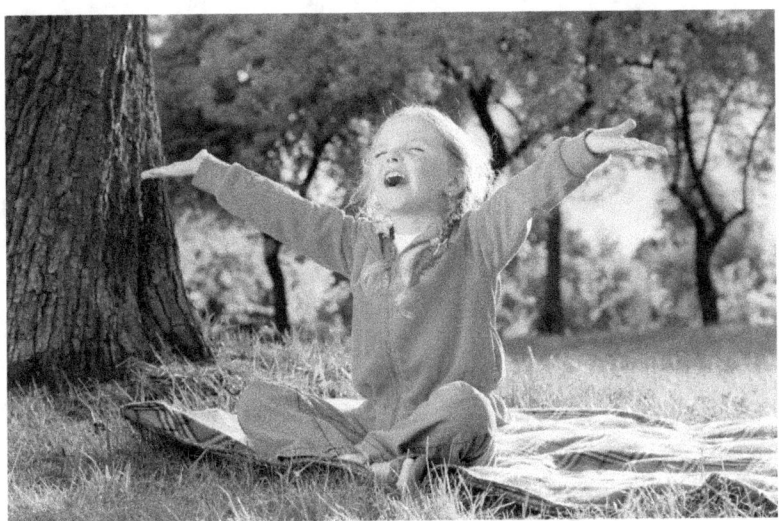

1)   Reduction of stress

The power of meditative mindfulness helps remove stress and relaxes the body. With the reduction of stress, the mind is at peace and can be more productive and happy.

2)   Elimination of depression

The power of yoga focuses on the positive and reduces anxiety and depression. The tools used to control depression are within the individual and can be brought to the fore, at will, any time.

3)   Better mental alertness

The improved breathing and increase in positive energy greatly increases mental alertness and concentration. Thus the individual is happier, more confident and in a better frame of mind to go about his/her daily routine.

Role of Yoga in Weight Loss

Let us first understand some of the causes which are responsible for the excess weight in the human body.

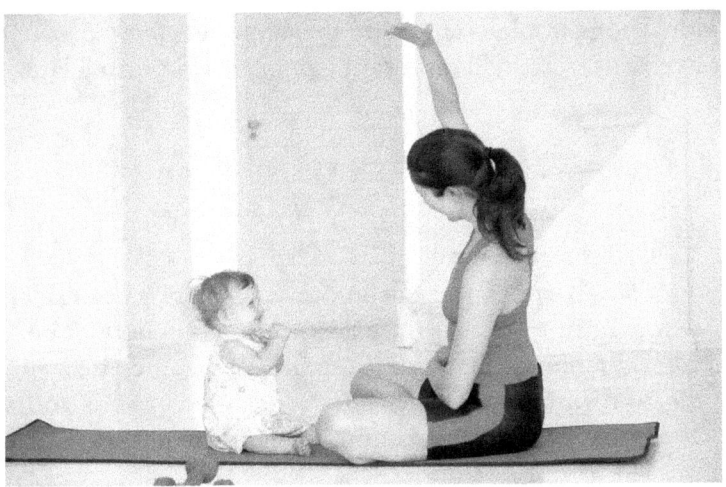

1)   Lifestyle

The human body is not designed for a sedentary lifestyle. Despite millions of years, our body's biology has not changed much. Our ancestors were hunters and gatherers, constantly on the move and alert for danger. If you take such a fit human body to sit behind a desk for 10 to 15 hours of the day, would it not revolt? The human body is designed for exercise and not a desk job. If we aren't going to be hunters and gatherers again, why not include some exercises into our lifestyle?

Most of us can't do aerobic exercises or visit a gym regularly. Reasons could vary from time constraint and lethargy to health problems like backaches, spondylosis and arthritis. With this step-by-step instructional yoga book, you can do the exercises on your own at your convenience. We will discuss the dos and don'ts in a later chapter.

2)   Hormonal changes

Hormones play an important role in our wellbeing. The endocrine glands secrete hormones that have a variety of functions. The optimum production of hormones establishes competent communication within the body. They affect your moods and emotions as well. Effective digestion, metabolism and excretion are also controlled by our hormones.

Yoga poses apply gentle pressure on the glands that pump hormones into our body. When one completes the pose, the pressure relaxes. This stimulates the sluggish glands and restores balance in its functioning. Yoga postures and breathing techniques bring about a balance in all our bodily functions. In some cases, weight gain could be a result of hormonal imbalances which can be improved through yoga.

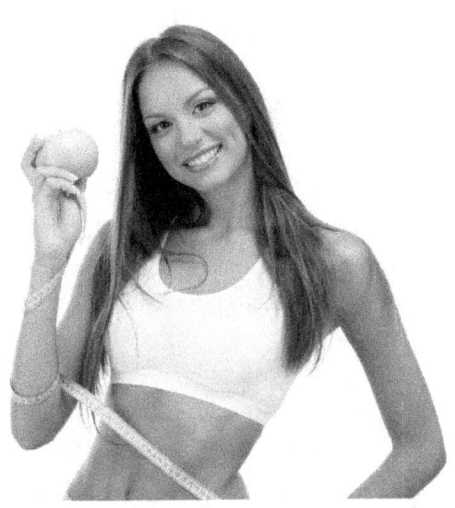

3) Dietary control

It is truly amazing that the mindfulness practice of yoga and its breathing techniques help strengthen the focus of your "inner eye." Also referred to as the "mind's eye," it helps make you watchful over what you eat, how you eat and where you eat. It disciplines your eating habits and thereby makes you a conscientious person.

4) Positive mindset

Diligent practice of yoga brings about greater positivity in your life. Your energy levels are high, facilitating exercise and you will get the drive to follow a healthier lifestyle. When you feel positive, you are happy and you spread happiness. When you see good results for your efforts, you will be passionate about all that you do.

There is no shortcut to success, but through yoga one will derive multiple benefits along the way! Isn't this what one can call "a great deal"?

Things to Prepare Before Getting Started with Yoga

Before every journey, one has to make some basic preparations. If you are attending a group class in a studio or park, you may like making adjustments accordingly. Let us now take a look at the things to keep in mind before we embark on this amazing journey.

1)   Fix a place and time

The venue where you are going to practice yoga is important. The place should be uncluttered and open. For indoors, choose a well ventilated and airy room. You will need a minimum floor space of 5 x 7 feet. Avoid places that are noisy with strong odors. Prefer no distraction while doing yoga. Soft, soothing music is fine. The floor should be even and non-skid. You don't want your mat moving around while you practice!

For an outdoor location, it should be a quiet place with no direct sunlight. Again, the surface should be smooth so you are not resting on any pebbles or creepy crawlies!

Assign a time for your yoga session. Early morning is the best time for yoga and try and be consistent.

2)   What to wear

Choose knee- or full-length athletic pants. For the top, wear closefitting clothes; you don't want the shirt rolling down over your head while working on the inverted poses! Depending on the weather, you may wear a long-sleeved T-shirt over a tank top. As you progress through the warm-up exercises, you may want to remove the outer layer.

Choose soft cotton fabric as you may break into a sweat. Cotton fabrics allow your skin to breathe. Avoid any obstructing jewellery and accessories.

Long hair should be tied up so that it doesn't fall on your face or eyes. The exercise is preferably done barefoot for proper balance. If required, snug-fitting socks may be worn.

Carry a towel to wipe off any excessive sweat.

3)   Eat and hydrate yourself

The last meal should be eaten at least 2 hours prior to the yoga session. Some forms of yoga may cause excessive perspiration, so drink sufficient amounts of fluids. Keep a bottle of water to sip from; visit the washroom before you begin to avoid breaks in-between. We'll discuss this further under the topic of "etiquette."

•   To get more out of yoga you need to eat and drink right. Gradually cut down or stop aerated drinks and caffeine intake. Eat more fresh fruits and raw vegetables. Limit the consumption of processed food or those with added preservatives.

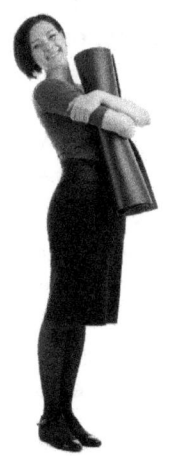

4)   A yoga mat

Yoga should not be done on the bare floor. A non-skid mat or carpet is recommended. For obvious reasons of hygiene, avoid sharing a mat. Some poses require you to lie face down so it is better to personalize your usage.

In the beginning, you need not worry about straps, bolsters or any such equipment. As you progress, you can gradually start using them.

5)   Be open

If you have any physical ailments or injuries, wait a while till the wound or muscle has healed. Check with your physician if you have any history of hypertension, high blood pressure or any heart condition. This will help decide what poses or breathing techniques you should avoid initially. Remember, that this is important as an incorrect posture or the use of inappropriate breathing techniques can cause more harm than good.

• Good to know

o   Have a wash up before you start the session.

o   Take a few minutes to settle down with your eyes closed and unwind. It also helps to slowly ease into the session. After a hectic day at work, you may not be able to switch gears immediately to the calmness required for yoga.

o   Remove your footwear outside the room, away from your mat.

o   Switch off your cell phone as you don't want to be disturbed and more importantly, a loud jingle in the midst of your meditation is not what you want.

o   Avoid perfumes/room fresheners as the breathing exercises may cause a heightened sense of smell.

o   Try not to fall asleep while doing the relaxation postures.

In the beginning, it may be a little challenging to keep up with the schedule. For many beginners it may be due to adjusting to the changes. Follow the three D's—discipline, determination and dedication—and very soon you will be glad to notice a great deal of improvement.

Over 30 Easy Poses for Beginners

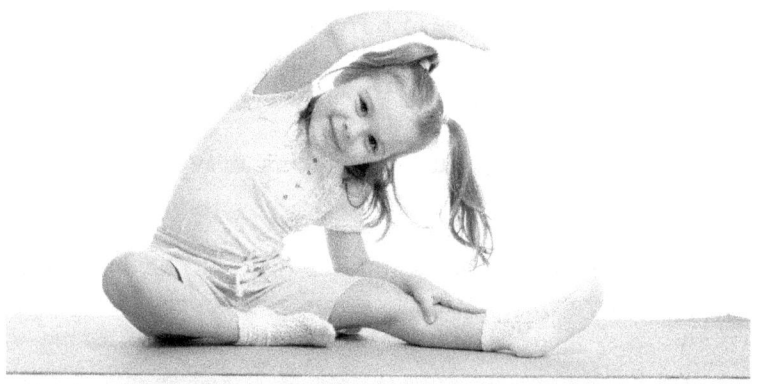

First and foremost, you need to set realistic goals.

Understand and respect your body. The role of genes and body type also determine body weight and ease in weight loss. Do not compare your flexibility with that of a fellow yoga practitioner. Each body differs and it is impossible to grow and improve if you are constantly comparing notes. The beauty of yoga is best experienced when you look from within. Respect your body and listen to it.

If you find it difficult to hold a particular pose, don't stretch it. It is fine if you can start with a 5-second hold. Gradually increase the time and before long you will soon be holding for a full minute! Do not expect quick results.

A Simpler, Easier and Faster Way to Weight Loss, Stress Relief, Heal Your Body and Find Inner Peace and Balance.

Do not wish for the moon. Be practical. While doing any pose, if you feel any discomfort or pain, come out of the pose and slowly unwind. Wait and watch for a few days before attempting it again.

As we are concentrating on weight loss, in this chapter we will learn poses that help weight loss along with hips, thighs, arms, and tummy toning.

Warming-up for Your Yoga Session

As with any form of exercise, it is important to warm-up before you commence and wind down at the end. On a physical level, it gears your body ready for the upcoming exercises and avoids the risk of injury. On a higher level, it makes the mind calmer and helps you focus inwards.

Yoga involves asanas(physical exercise) and praanayaam (control of life force, meaning breath). It is vital to focus on both simultaneously. Great importance is placed on pranayaam in yoga. It also plays a central role in meditation. As you read, you will notice that the asanas are catered to every age and body type.

We will discuss some warming-up exercises many of which can be done even while watching the television or cooking. Now that you have taken this step forward, keep your muscles moving. Flex your legs, shoulders, neck and back muscles as often as possible, especially if you have a sedentary job.

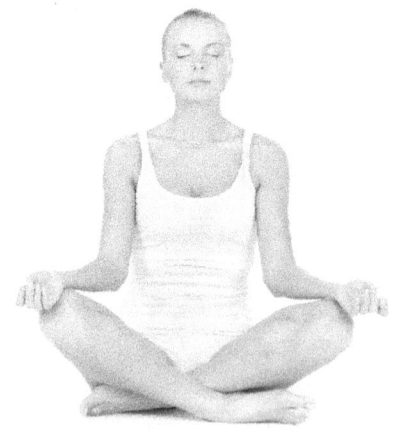

•   Sitting posture

Sit on the mat with legs crossed.

This pose is traditionally known as sukhaasan [*Ease pose*].

It is very beneficial for the body.

A higher form of this is padmaasana [*Lotus pose*]. This is done with each foot over the opposite thigh. This helps digestion and controls blood pressure. A variation can be with done by placing one foot over the opposite thigh.

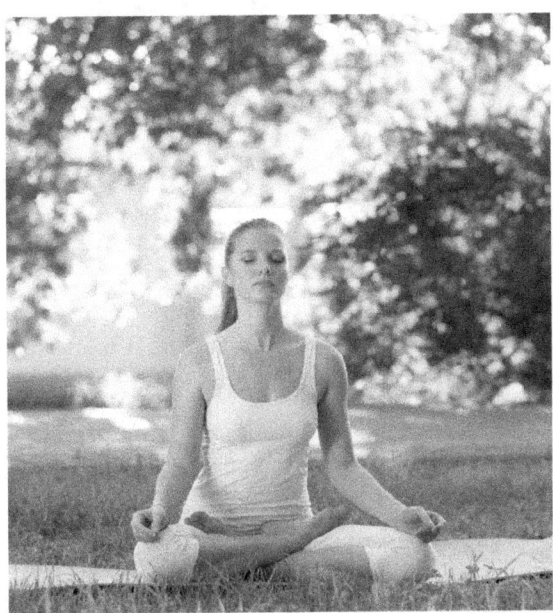

Gradually, your flexibility will improve and you will be more comfortable sitting in this pose.

It will take a few days to improve flexibility. Eventually the aim is to sit for longer stretches of time in sukhaasan.

Important note: Spine must be erect, shoulders back and relaxed, chin slightly lifted for ease in breathing.

This is a simple, yet highly beneficial posture.

Contraindications: People with joint pain and any knee/ankle injuries should avoid this pose.

A Simpler, Easier and Faster Way to Weight Loss, Stress Relief, Heal Your Body and Find Inner Peace and Balance.

• **Close your eyes.** Many asanas are done with eyes closed to improve concentration and to avoid distraction.

Important note: You may feel tempted to keep your eyes open, however don't fight the urge. Go with the flow. Try by closing your eyes for 10 breaths. As the days progress, increase the count by 5 per day till you can sit with eyes closed for 3 to 4 minutes.

• **Observe your breath.** Pranayaam involves the extension of life-giving breath. Observe how you breathe. It is most likely shallow and there is an expansion of the chest cavity. Try to take deeper breaths. Place your right palm on your abdomen. As you breathe in, expand the abdomen and feel it rise. This way all the lobes of the lungs work and function to the fullest.

Important note: Avoid straining while you breathe. It must be as silent as a regular breath. Just focus on expanding the abdomen while inhaling and contracting while exhaling. It should be like the breathing of a sleeping baby. As we aged, we incorrectly reduce the intensity of our breath which causes problems.

Do abdominal breathing for 12 sets. An inhalation and exhalation comprises 1 set.

The 5 Basic Movements of Yoga

- ## Neck Movements [KanthaSanchalana]

1)   Slowly, turn your head towards the left reaching as far back towards your shoulder as comfortably possible.

Breathe in as you turn and breathe out as you face the front. In the same gentle manner, turn to the right.

Follow the same breathing pattern. Feel the stretch in the neck muscles.

Repeat 4 times on each side. Hold in position for 4 breaths.

2)   Breathe in and raise your head towards the ceiling.

Breathe out and gently bring it down, chin touching the chest.

Repeat for 4 counts. Hold in position for 4 breaths.

Contraindications: If you have a history of spondylosis, do check with your physician before you attempt this.

Objective: To improve the stamina and flexibility of our neck muscles.

- ## Shoulder Movements [SkandhaSanchalana]

1) Sit in Ease pose. Place your fingers on your shoulders.

Draw imaginary circles with your elbows.

Get them to make large circular movements.

Feel the movement of your shoulder blades.

Be sure that the movements are slow and exaggerated.

Make your elbows touch in the front.

Do 4 circles clockwise and 4 counter-clockwise.

2) Raise your arms in front of you. Do not keep them stiff.

Fold your fingers into a fist with the thumbs inside.

Rotate the wrist in a figure 8.

Do this for 6 counts. Reverse the movement for another 6 counts.

Relax with eyes closed for 4 breaths.

Rest with hands on your knees and palms facing upwards and keep your eyes closed.

Feel the tension drain from the shoulder and neck region.

Objective: To help strengthen our stamina and flexibility of our neck and shoulder muscles; especially helpful for practitioners with backaches.

• ## Hand Movements [HastaSanchalana]

1)   In lying down position, place your hands by your sides, legs apart.

Lift your hands slightly above ground. Keeping your arms straight, slowly swing both hands towards your head, parallel to the ground till the 2 palms meet. Place one palm on the other.

Stretch your hands in the upward direction and your legs in the downward direction for about 10 seconds.

Return to the original position by the same path in slow motion.

Important note: The movements are to be done in a slow and continuous motion; hands are to be kept straight and avoid bending at the elbows while doing the exercise.

Objective: To enhance the stamina and flexibility for muscles around the neck and shoulder.

• Leg Movements [PadaSanchalana]

1)   Stay seated but stretch your legs in front of you. Keep your feet a little apart.

Place your hands on your thighs or on the mat on the side of your hips.

Twist the feet inwards so the toes touch each other.

Then twist them outwards as far down as you can so the side of the foot touches the ground.

Repeat 10 times.

2)   In lying down relax position, place your hands by your sides, legs apart.

Move both hands slowly towards your head, bend at elbows to place the hands around your head resting on the ground.

Lift up the left leg and move it near your hip. Repeat the same procedure for your right leg.

End by slowly returning both hands back to the sides of your body.

Important note: The movements are to be done in a slow and continuous motion. Do not strain your body during the exercise.

Objective: To increase our strength and flexibility of muscles around our legs, hips and hip joints.

- ## Knee Movements [JanuSanchalana]

1)   In lying down facing up position, similar to the leg movement exercise, place your hands by your sides, legs apart.

Move both hands slowly towards your head, bend at elbows to place the hands around your head, resting on the ground.

Bend at your left knee and place the left foot close to your hips, then turn the left knee to the right side as much as you can.

Repeat the same steps above for your right leg.

End by slowly returning both hands back to the sides of your body.

2)   Lying down facing up, place hands around your head, resting on the ground.

Bending both legs at the knees, bring both feet close to your hips.

Turn both knees to the left side as much as possible.

While touching the ground with your left knee, turn your head to the right side.

Breathe normally and relax all your muscles.

End by slowly returning both legs and hands back to the original position.

Important note: The movements are to be done in a slow and continuous motion. Do not strain your body during the exercise.

Objective: To aid the strengthening and flexibility of our muscles at our waist, knees, joints at the hips and knees, and our spinal column.

Now that you are geared up and ready, let's get started with our weight loss exercise!

12 Efficacious Yoga Poses for Weight Loss

Loss of muscle tone, stress and anxiety are often accompanied by weight gain. They could be a cause or a result of the excess weight. To successfully address weight loss, we must use a multiple approach to overcome it.

Sun Salutation [Surya Namaskar]

Surya namaskar is one set of the most powerful and comprehensive exercises in yoga for beginners. Being done at a slow pace helps improve your stamina and flexibility. Once you learn the sequence of the 12 asanas well, the speed and energy can increase and will work as a cardiovascular exercise. While the postures increase your awareness of your body, the breathing pattern involved here stimulates your energy levels.

Step 1: Prayer pose [Pranamasana]

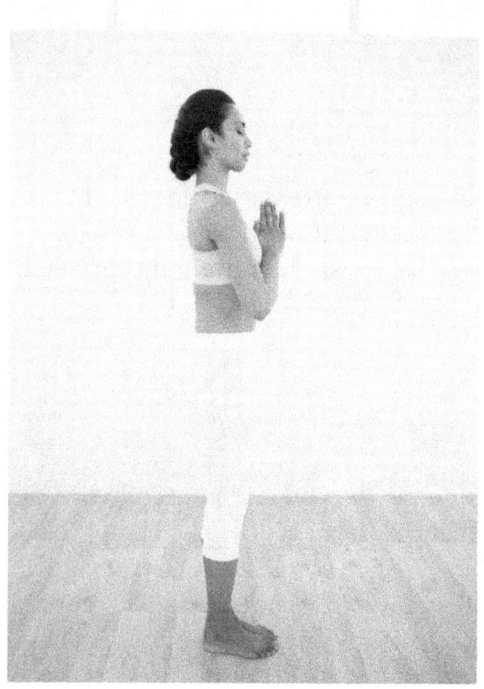

•   Position yourself to begin by standing firmly on the ground.

•   Expand your chest and relax your shoulders.

•   Inhale and as you exhale, bring palms together in front of your chest in a prayer pose.

Step 2: Raised hands pose [UrdhvaHastasana]

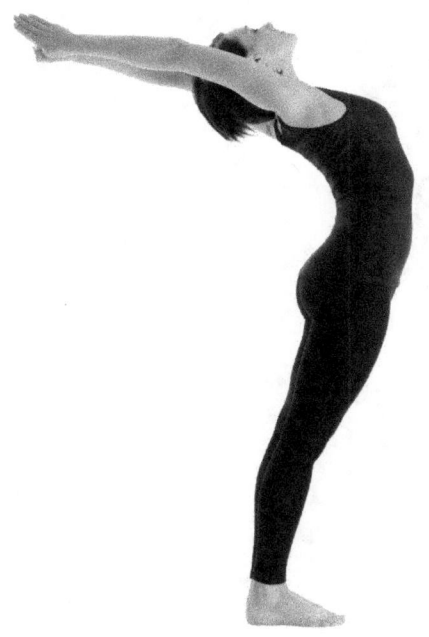

- Inhale and raise your arms above your head.

- Ensure your biceps touch your ears.

- Tilt the body backwards slightly but try to concentrate on the elongation of the pose.

Step 3: Hand to foot pose [Padahastasana]

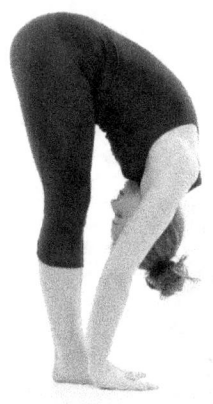

•   Breathe out normally and gently bend forward to place your palms on either side of your feet.

•   You may bend your knees if needed.

•   Try not to shift the position of your palms till the completion of the entire sequence.

Step 4: Equestrian or Horse stance pose [Ashwasanchalanasana]

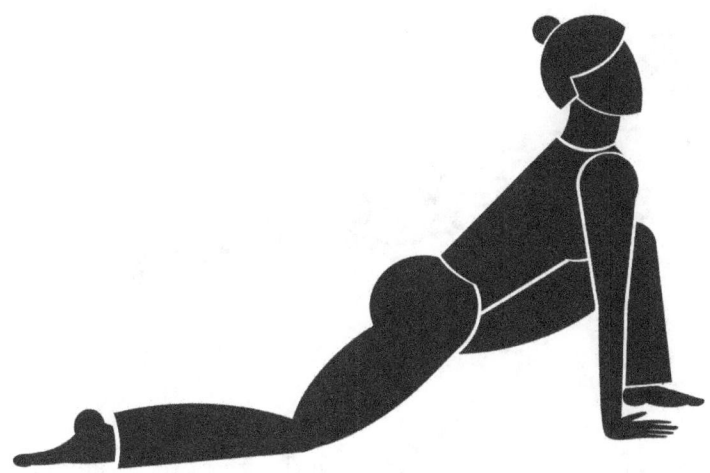

•	In squatting down position, breathe in and push the right leg back resting on the toes with your knee touching the floor.

•	Raise your head.

•	Keep your arms straight with palms touching the mat as your support. Bend your left knee and place the left foot in between your palms.

•	Erect the foot position behind you and bring the bending knee backwards to prepare for the plank pose.

Step 5: Plank pose [Uttihitachaturangadandasana]

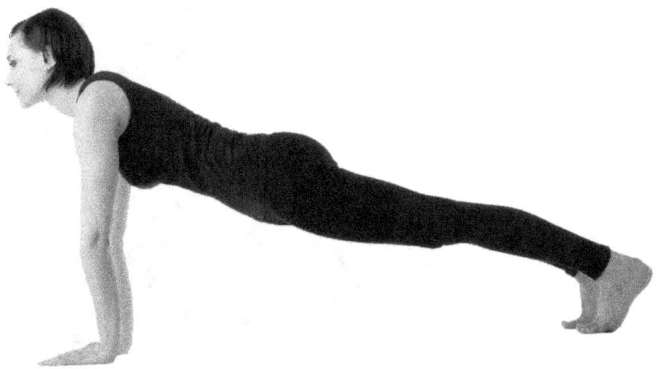

- Exhale and move the left leg behind with both legs extended.

- Neck, spine and legs are in one straight line.

- Arms should be perpendicular to the floor.

- Weight is evenly distributed over hands and toes.

- Inhale bring your knees down and forehead to the floor.

- Sit on your calves, like in child pose. (You may refer to child pose image in future chapter.)

- Take a few breaths and relax your arms.

Step 6: Eight point salutation [Ashtanganamaskara]

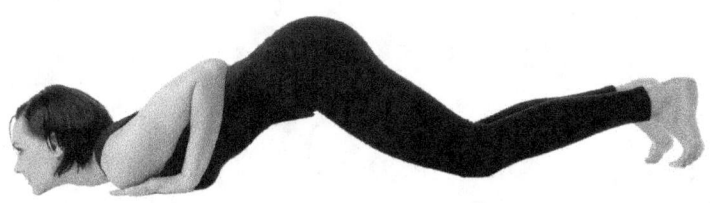

As the name of the pose denotes, eight parts of the body touch the ground: chin, chest, 2 hands, 2 knees and 2 feet.

•   Inhale and stretch forward (as in step 5) but bend your arms at the elbows.

•   You are almost prone on your belly.

•   Raise your hips from the floor.

Step 7: Cobra pose [Bhujangasana]

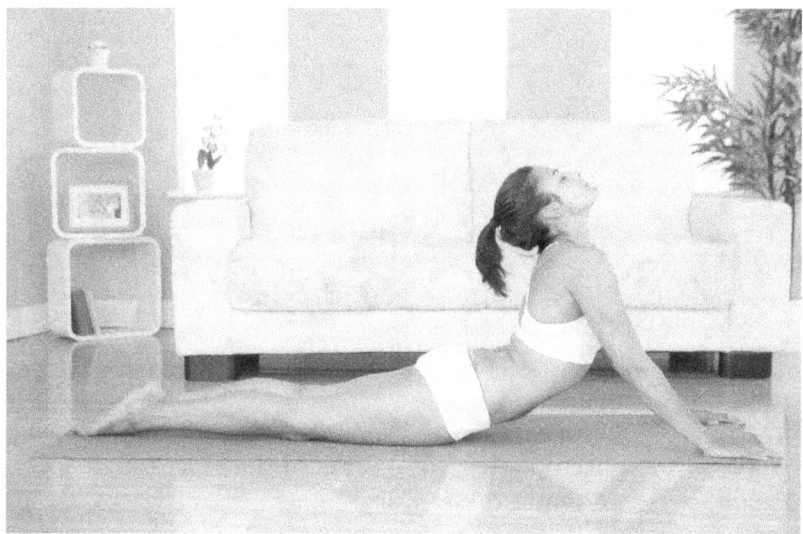

•   As you inhale, raise your head and push the upper body upwards.

•   Arms can be slightly bent but hips are on the floor.

•   Get off your toes and relax your feet.

Step 8: Downward Dog Pose [AdhoMukhaSvanasana]

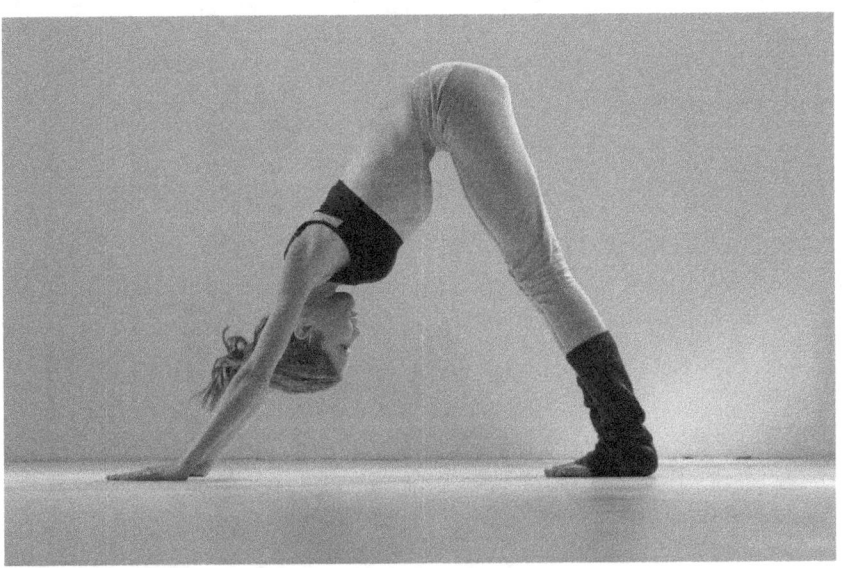

• As you exhale, place your feet flat on the mat and raise your hips forming an inverted 'V'.

• Keep your head parallel to your straightened arms.

• Try to keep your heels flat on the floor at all times. (*Different from the Dog Pose described in the later pages)

• Erect your feet, bend your knees and lower your hips to release from position.

Step 9: Equestrian pose [Ashwasanchalanasana]

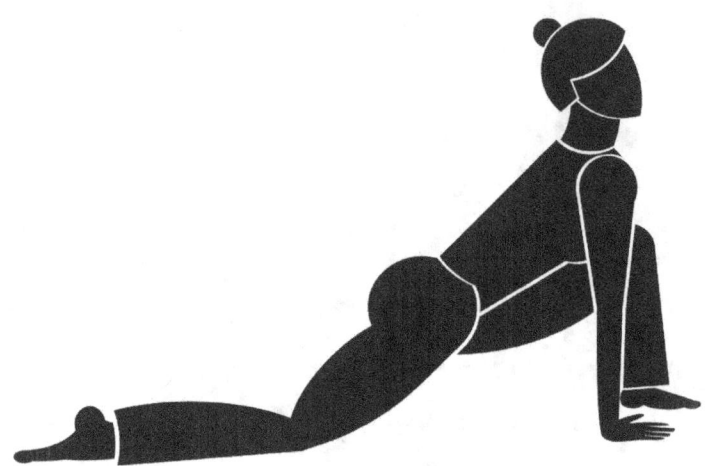

- Breathe in and bring your left foot to the front.

- Try to reach it to a spot between your palms.

- If not, don't worry, with practice you will soon be able to!

- Raise your head up and push your hips down.

- Bring both legs to squatting position to release from pose.

Step 10: Hand to foot pose [Padahastasana]

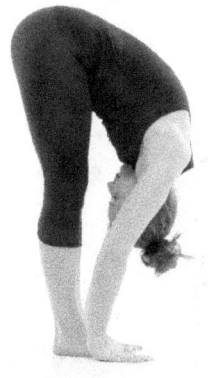

- Breathe out and bring your 2 feet together.

- Try not to move the palms.

- Bend your knees if required.

Step 11: Raised hands pose [Urdhvahastasana]

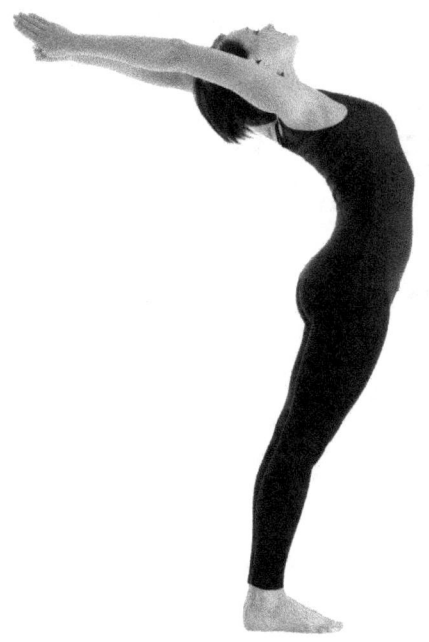

• Breathe in slowly and gently raise your head, rolling up one vertebra at a time.

• With arms staying along the side of your head, raise your body.

• Gently bend backward, maintaining your balance.

Step 12: Prayer pose [Pranamasana]

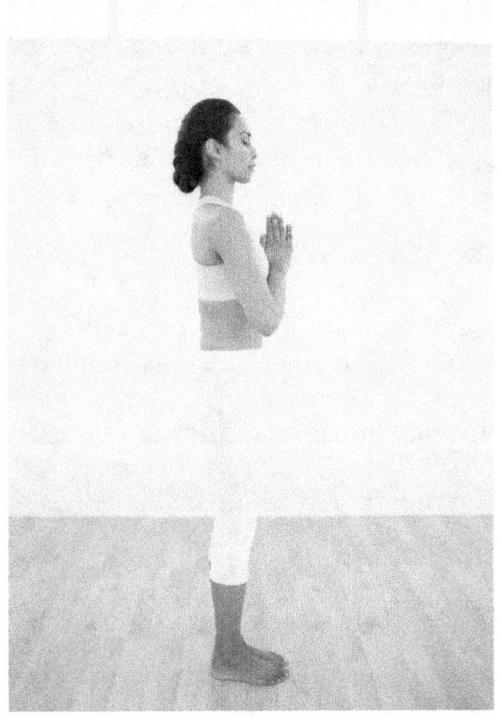

•   Exhale and straighten up with arms still raised.

•   Slowly lower the arms down in a wide arc and join your palms in a prayer pose.

•   These 12 steps complete one round.

•   Two rounds make up one set.

•   For the second round, follow the same instructions.

- The only variation being between step 4 and 10 starting with the right leg instead of the left.

- Stand with feet shoulder-width apart and eyes closed.

Closely observe your breathing pattern and to the sensations of your body.

Stay in this position for about 20 breaths.

- Lie down with feet wide apart and arms on the side with palms facing up and eyes closed. Observe your body's sensation.

Remain in lying down position till your heartbeat returns to normal.

Slowly, turn onto your right side, bring your knees up and hug them tight. Imagine you are in a fetus stage, safe and secure.

Hold for 30 seconds and release.

- Place your left palm on the mat near the right shoulder and push yourself up to a seated position, keeping eyes closed.

Rub your palms together briskly to generate some heat. Place them gently over your eyes.

Hold for 10 seconds and open your eyes.

Welcome back! You have returned rejuvenated!

Points to note

☐   Sun salutations are most effective when done on an empty stomach early in the morning.

☐   This exercise should always be done in even numbers—one round with the left leg and then with the right. Start with one set and then gradually increase the quantity as you wish.

☐   Closely observe your body's reaction to differentiate the difference between good pain (due to stiffness) and bad pain (due to injury).

Contraindications: Learners who suffer from hypertension, high blood pressure, have a heart condition or have had a recent abdominal surgery should consult a physician before doing these poses.

Objective: To shake off the extra fat on the belly, lose extra calories and keep you naturally in the proper shape you desire. Gradually try aiming for 32 rounds of sun salutation poses to be done in 8 minutes per day!

This set of 12 poses serves as a good link between the warm-up exercises and the yoga poses coming up in the next few pages. Let's move on to explore more!

Simple and Effective Yoga Poses for Trimming 'That' Waistline

Triangle pose [Trikonaasana]

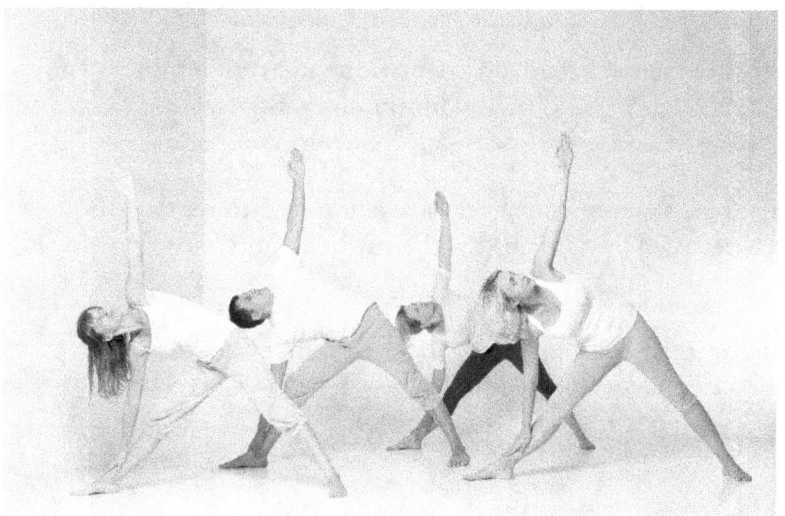

• Stand with feet spread wide apart and firmly planted on the ground. Position your right foot parallel to your shoulder while the left foot should be pointing straight forward in 90-degrees to your left foot heels.

• Bring your arms parallel to the ground. Keep your right hand close to your right ankle as you bring your left hand above your head.

• Look up at your left hand pointing to the ceiling. Hold this pose for at least a minute with regular breathing.

•   Switch sides by returning your body to upright position and exchange your feet's pointing directions.

•   Lower the left hand to the left ankle and look up at your right hand.

•   Do this for two rounds. Return to standing posture and relax.

Contraindications: These exercises are to be avoided during pregnancy and soon after abdominal surgery. To be also avoided by those who have a spinal injury, slipped disc, hernia, migraine, high blood pressure or diarrhea.

Objective: To aid in maintaining proper body balance, strengthening of leg muscles and removes fat accumulated around the waist section. It helps enhance the digestive system, nervous system and reproductive organs. Thus it also gives therapeutic benefits to practioners with digestive problems, constipation and depression.

Sitting Half Spinal Twist [Ardhmatsyendrasana]

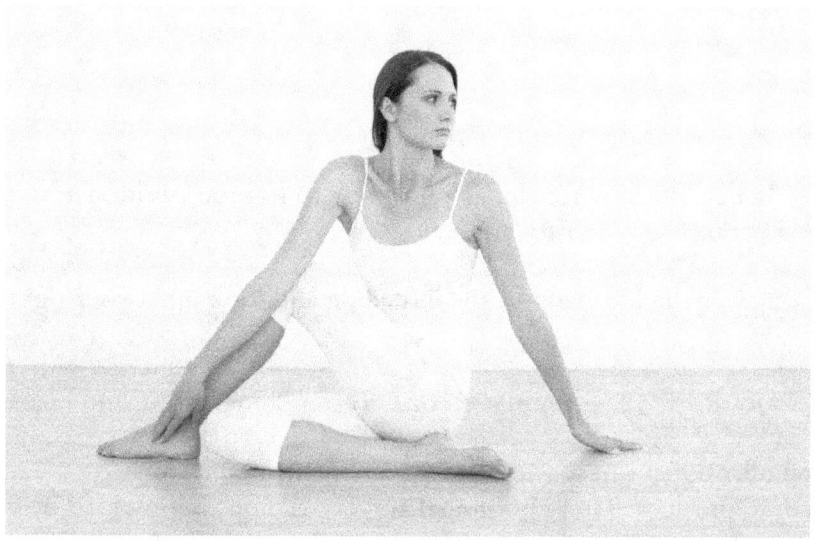

•　　Sit on the mat with spine erect and legs stretched out. Place feet together.

•　　Bend your right leg and place that foot near the left hip.

•　　Bend your left leg and place it over the right leg near the right knee.

•　　Place your right hand on the left ankle, and place your right hand on the mat behind you. Hold this pose for a few regular breaths.

•　　As you exhale, turn around and straighten the legs. Repeat on the other side. One set a day.

•　　Relax with eyes closed.

Objective: To tone up the round shoulders, reduce the appetite and improve constipation as more digestive juices is produced from the abdominal organs. It helps release the tension accumulated in the arms, shoulders, neck and upper back area. This pose is useful for a slipped disc and relieving stiffness and back pain between the vertebrae.

It is also beneficial to women's reproductive organs and urinary system as well as menstrual disorders.

Quick and Useful Yoga Poses for Achieving a Sexy Flat Tummy

A major region of worry for overweight people is the tummy. Well, a simple yoga exercise will help improve the muscle tone.

Leg raise [Uttanapadasana]

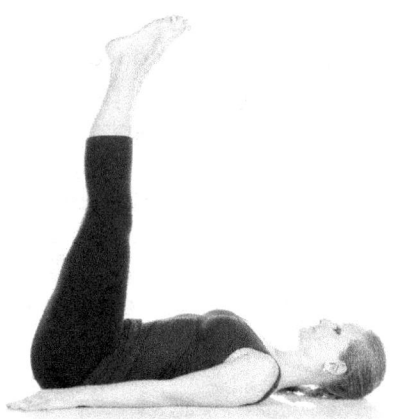

- Lie down on the mat and focus on the tummy area

- Place your hands under your tail bone for support. Tighten the abdomen.

- Inhale and raise one leg from the floor to a 90-degree angle.

- Exhale and bring it down. See that the neck is not arched and that the back is flat on the ground.

- Do this for both legs.

• Increasing the difficulty level will be to raise the leg to 45 degrees and to hold in position for a few seconds.

• The next level will involve lifting both legs together. First to 90 degrees and then to 45 degrees, hold in that position for a few seconds.

Always follow this with the reverse exercise by lying down on your stomach and lifting the leg backwards for a few counts.

Contraindications: Learners with backaches can avoid holding this pose. It can be done without holding at the raised position.

Variation of Uttanapadasana

Lie down with arms raised above your head. Lift the leg to 90 degrees and raise the upper body too. Touch the hands to the legs and return to the prone position. Start with 4counts and go up to 12.

Objective: To tone up and strengthen the muscles at the thigh, hamstrings, abdominal lower back and pelvic area. This exercise facilitates removal of constipation and flatulence. It is beneficial for practitioners with lower back pain.

Boat Pose [Navasana]

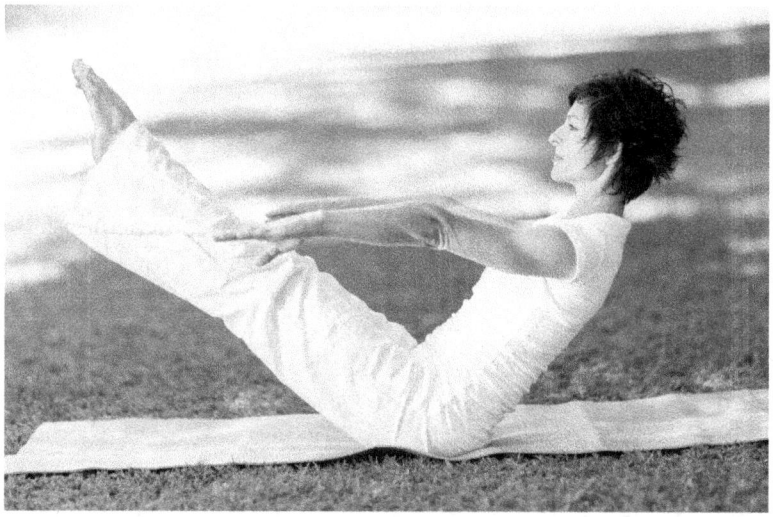

• Lie down on your back. Place arms by your side and put your feet together.

• Inhale deeply and as you exhale, lift your upper body and arms towards your legs. Simultaneously lift the legs a few inches off the ground.

• Breathe deeply while you hold this pose.

• Relax and return to the starting pose. Repeat 6 times.

Objective: To enhance the toning of your thigh, calf and abdominal muscles, thereby reducing fat around the abdominal section. The boat pose creates pressure that not only improves the function of our kidneys, liver, pancreas and intestines but also the blood circulation of our legs. It subsides nervous tension, after which gives the practitioner a refreshing, energizing and positive feel.

Cat-cow stretch Pose [chakravakasana]

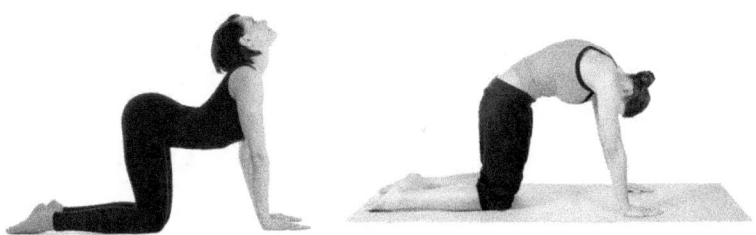

• Begin in a table top position, with arms (shoulder-width apart) and knees apart like 4 legs of a table in perpendicular to the shoulders and hips respectively. Hands and feet flat on the mat.

• Breathe out long and curve up your spine (flexion) pointing it towards the ceiling, while maintaining your knees and shoulders stationery.

• Breathe in and release tension on your spine to return to straight back.

• Maintaining in table top position, breathe in deeply and arch your spine (extension) down towards the floor direction. Perform the poses in slow motions in conjunction with deep breaths and continue till your spine feels relaxed.

Contraindications: If you have a neck injury or a spine medical history, you may like to avoid this pose or consult a doctor before performing it.

Objective: To strengthen the tummy muscles and functions of your belly organs. This exercise calms your mind, aids in your stretch of the neck, back and torso and at the same time massages the spine and its muscles. It is beneficial for practitioners with reproductive concerns.

Easy Yoga Poses to get your Arms and Thighs into Shape

Most of the poses when held for a few minutes can strengthen the muscles.

Warrior Pose I [Veerabhadrasana I]

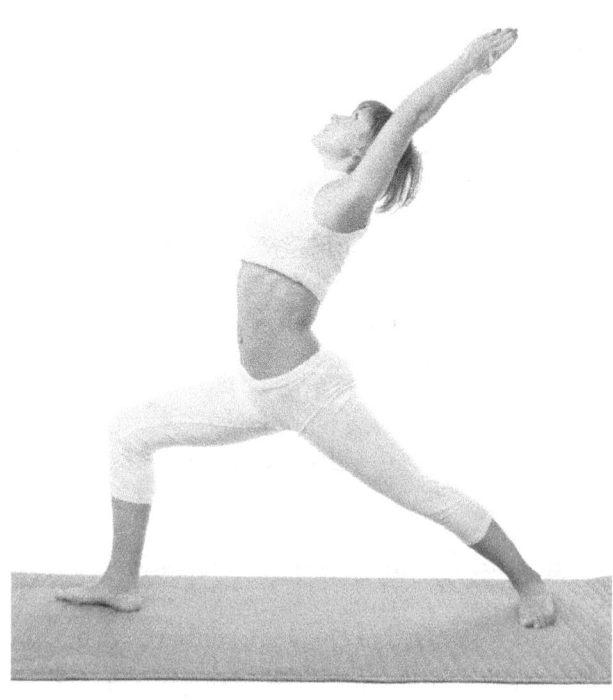

- Stand with feet wide apart. Turn the right foot with toes pointing to the right. Turn your left foot slightly inwards in a 45 degree position.

- Raise the arms above the head. Turn your body to face the right side. Bend the right leg slightly at the knee.

- The bent knee should not be positioned beyond the right foot.

- Hold this posture for a few minutes focusing on a spot to maintain balance. Feel the tightening in the thigh. Breathe normally.

- Return to start pose by turning the toes to the front.

- Repeat for the left side.

Objective: To drain fat away from the abdominal area and to tone up and strengthen the legs and abdomen. The warrior pose exercise enhances blood flow to our joints at the ankles, knee, hips and shoulders. It is also beneficial for the coordination between our musculoskeletal and nervous system thus maintaining a well-balanced body!

Dog Pose [AdhoMukhaSvanasana]

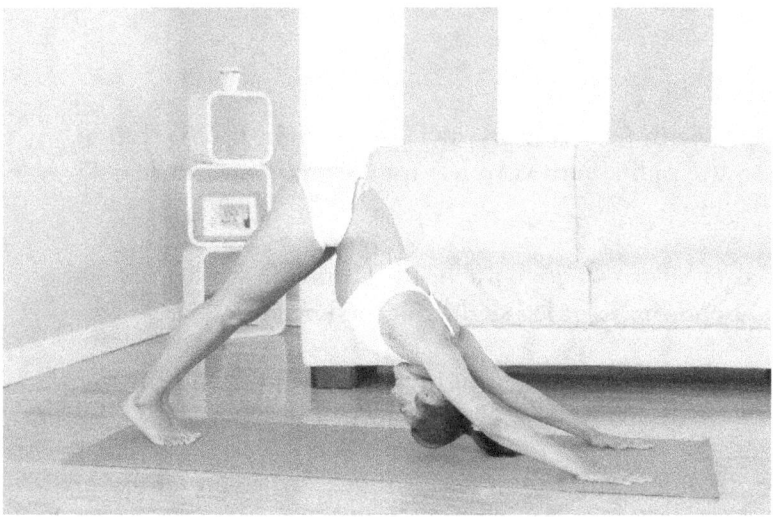

• Start in a table top position, with arms (shoulder-width apart) and knees apart like 4 legs of a table. Keep your hands with your fingers gripping the mat and heels erected with the toes on the mat.

• Prepare to rise by first taking a breath in, and while breathing out, raise your hips and push your body backwards followed by lowering your heels onto the mat. Ensure both your neck and your back are in a straight line.

• Hold in position for 4 long, deep breaths.

• Prepare to release the position by first taking a breath in and while breathing out, gradually lower your hips and knees to return back to a table top position. Relax.

Contraindications: Learners with heart ailments, migraine and high blood pressure should avoid this pose.

Objective: To burn fat from the waist section and give a good shape to our arms and legs. This exercise energizes our body by relieving the feeling of exhaustion, fatigue, stiffness and pain in the shoulder blades and heels. It is beneficial for practitioners with low blood pressure and anyone who wishes to have their brain cells refreshed.

Try working on this posture for a few attempts. Do you feel lighter in your legs, heels and ankles?

Cobbler's Pose [BaddhaKonasana]

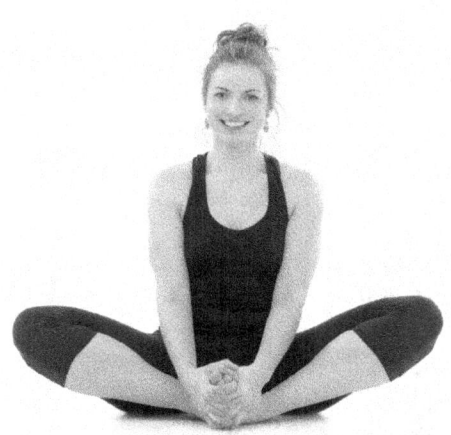

- Sit up straight with knees bent, soles gently pressing against one another and both hands holding your feet or toes (you may hold on to your lower leg if you wish in the beginning).

- Breathe out and bring your heels as close to your body as possible, avoid straining your knees. Maintain a tall, straight back posture and focus on your breathing. Hold in position for 1–5 minutes.

- Breathe in and return to original sitting position.

Objective: To stretch and strengthen the inner thighs, knees and groin areas. The cobbler's pose aids removal of fatigue and anxiety. It is beneficial for practitioners with flat feet, infertility, asthma and high blood pressure.

Bust the Stress and...Relax Yoga Poses

Child Pose [Balasana]

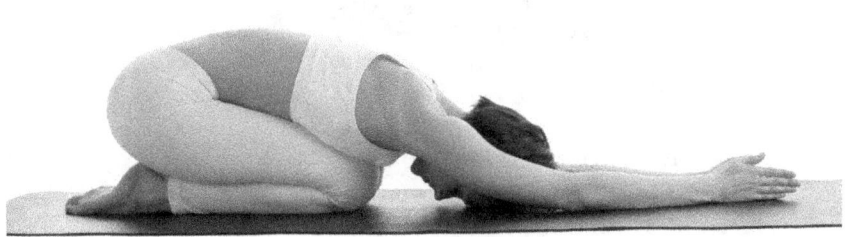

•   Sit on your calves with feet flat on the floor.

•   Bend forward and stretch the arms on the ground. Relax the arms and back.

•   Sink into the pose and feel the tension drain away. Breathe long and deep. Stay in this pose for about 2–3 minutes.

•   Get up slowly, one vertebra at a time.

Objective: To stretch and strengthen the thighs, ankles and hips muscles. The child pose asana tranquilizes the mind and relieves tension and stress. It is beneficial for anger management.

Upward Dog Pose [UrdhvaMukhaShvanasana]

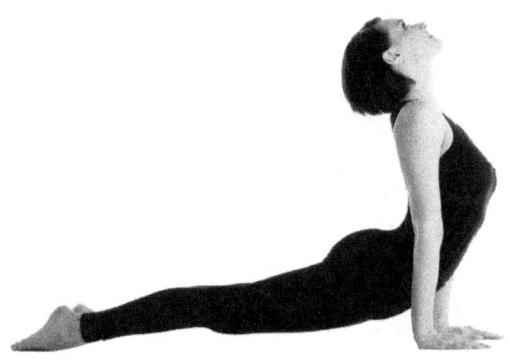

- Lie down on your mat face down.

- Place palms on both sides of the chest.

- Push yourself all the way up and straighten your arms. (*Different from the cobra pose as the arms are held straight and perpendicular to the floor with the legs and pelvis lifted off the ground.)

- Tilt the head back and breathe. Experience a sense of peace.

- Hold for 6–10 seconds.

- Release your position slowly and relax.

Objective: To expand the chest and refresh the spine. The upward dog pose facilitates the removal of constipation and flatulence. It is beneficial for practitioners with stiff back, backache, lower back pain and slipped disc.

Corpse Pose [Shavasana]

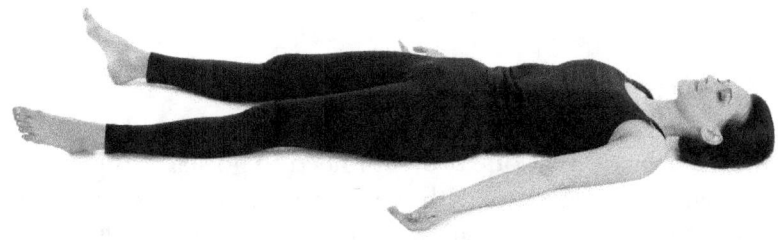

• Lie on your back, feet slightly apart and arms loosely placed on the sides, palms up.

• Close your eyes and let your feet hang limp.

• Start from your toes and switch off all the tension as you proceed to the top of your head.

• Take a deep breath and relax as you exhale. Imagine a calm and serene place within you. Lose yourself in its beauty. Breathe normally.

Objective: To relax the nervous system, entire body, muscles and mind. This exercise calms the mind, subsides stress and fatigue and improves our conscious and unconscious awareness. It is beneficial for practitioners with stress-related ailments, high blood pressure and insomnia.

Finding Inner Peace

The beauty of yoga is that one does not need to go searching for peace and happiness. It exists within our soul. All we have to do is look within. Yoga's simple breathing patterns promote good health of mind and body. Through breathing and mindful practices, one can unlock inner peace. It takes you to a place away from the worries and stress of life.

Regular practice of exercise, breathing and mindfulness will make you love yourself more than ever before. You will learn to accept yourself with greater calmness and face the trials of daily life with confidence.

Through yoga, one is in complete control of emotions which brings serenity.

Yoga, Meditation and Mindfulness—Mapping the Connection

As discussed earlier, yoga bridges the gap between body, mind and spirit. Through the practice of yoga, one develops a finer sense of that connection. The negative emotions that surface are quelled and replaced with positive ones. One enjoys better health both physically and mentally. Mindfulness involves changing our response to something beyond our control.

The silent power of mindfulness cannot be ignored. By focusing on the task or activity without any disturbances or judgement, one attains optimum results. The essence of yoga is to derive the power of concentration. Once you are able to focus on something, the efficiency of the job done is high. You are able to handle any form of crisis at work or home. You are able to bring clarity into your thoughts to resolve issues. Nothing will seem impossible. You will positively radiate the energy, develop empathy and communicate effectively.

Using the benefits of yoga and mindfulness, the much higher level of meditation will be easier to achieve. Meditation involves concentrating on your breath to transcend any ego and find your inner divinity. We realize our greater sense of purpose and are able to see things and observe actions more objectively.

However, to attain this level of connection does take time, dedication and discipline. The mastery over yoga is the stepping stone to the higher aspects of mindfulness and meditation.

Stay Focus and Track Your Success

As with any form of exercise, persistence pays. Weight gain, being a complicated process, will take time and effort to overcome. Many people are tempted to try quick-fix solutions for weight loss. Not only is it impossible, it is downright dangerous to put your precious body through that ordeal.

Be positive and love yourself. You are a special person, beautiful inside and out. Throw all the criticism away and stay focused on developing yoga as a way of life! Remember that you are a strong individual who will overcome all odds.

An important point to remember is that you must learn to tune in to your body. Listen to it. If you are feeling a "bad pain" in your back, then do not "hold" the leg raise exercise. Do gentle lifts for a few days till the pain subsides. Do the back strengthening Cobra pose. Yet another plus point is that of the hundreds of asanas, there is always something you can do. After mastering the exercises in this book for beginners, it is hoped that you will progress towards widening your knowledge.

The effect of yoga postures last for about 20–24 hours. So it is a good idea to do at least a few asanas every day. Try planning out a schedule to attempt longer sessions on some days. You can even split it between morning and evening.

Keep track of your progress. It may be disappointing if you are unable to do all the poses. But make a note of how many counts of each you are able to do. Take it from there. The optimum plan to lose weight is when you can do many rounds of sun salutations with intensity and speed. Combine yoga with plenty of fluids, a good diet and a healthier lifestyle. Include brisk walks in your schedule. A good idea is to try to get a companion to do yoga with; you will be sharing goodness.

Conclusion

It takes many years to perfect the postures and breathing techniques and the practice of mindfulness. Yoga enthusiasts the world over will vouch for the fact that they cannot skip even a single day's practice. If you are regular with the exercises, your muscle tone will definitely improve, giving you a better posture and appearance. Use yoga to unlock the intelligence of your body.

Be patient and you will see positive results. You will develop better self-esteem and your confidence will soar! Through yoga, you gain inner strength to make intelligent food choices and an improved lifestyle. Thus, you are tripling the benefits! Through the improvement in fitness, your sleep pattern will improve. The good functioning of your organs will help improve metabolism and you will feel rejuvenated. Your thoughts indicate who you are. So fill them with goodness.

It is true that slow and steady wins the race. Be mindful of your thoughts and actions and get the most out of life!

~ Lake Hills

Claim Your Freebie

Congratulations to you in completing reading your book. To claim your freebie, simply send an email stating your name, title and author of the book which you have purchased to: lakehillshub@gmail.com and we will revert to you with your freebie to help you kick-start your healthy living lifestyle!

Check Out Other Books

Below you'll find some of the other popular books that are popular on Amazon and Kindle as well. Simply click on the links below to check them out.

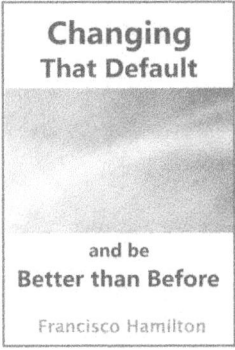

Changing That Default And Be Better Than Before

http://www.amazon.com/dp/B0105OYJLG

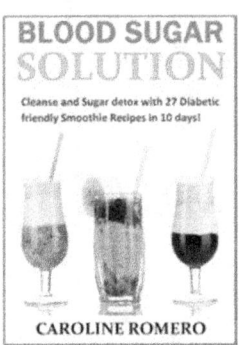

Blood Sugar Solution: Cleanse and Sugar detox with 27 Diabetic friendly Smoothie Recipes in 10 days!

http://www.amazon.com/dp/B00ZAP56AE

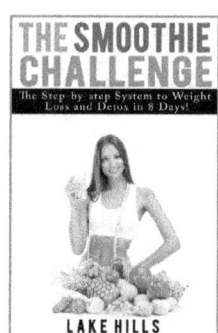

The Smoothie Challenge: The Step-by-step System to Weight Loss and Detox in 8 Days!

http://www.amazon.com/dp/B00XJS232I

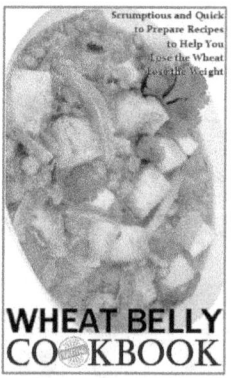

Wheat Belly Cookbook: 53 Scrumptious and Quick to Prepare Recipes to Help You Lose the Wheat Lose the Weight

http://www.amazon.com/dp/B00XXULZ7Q